I0696033

BEST

SOLUTION TO

DIABETES

DEDICATED TO

ALL

LIVING SOUL

<u>*ACKNOWLEDGEMENT*</u>

All praise and adoration is due to nobody except almighty God

the lord of mankind. I praise him and glorified him for is

protections and blessings over me so far. And also for giving me

opportunities to create this small work, for the benefit of my

readers. I am also indebted to my late father for his

tremendous efforts to make my education successful. May his

gentle soul continue to rest in perfect peace till eternity

(amen). And also to my great mother for her intensive supports

on every steps I take. May she live long to eat the fruit of her labor. This work would not have seen the light of the day if not

for the prayers, patronage and encouragement of my readers. I

thank you all, may almighty God in his infinity mercy continue

to bless and protect every one of us (amen).

CONTENTS

<u>**Section 1**</u>: Prologue to Diabetes

Diabetes is an ongoing infection that influences a large number of

individuals around the world. It is described by elevated degrees of

sugar (glucose) in the blood, either in light of the fact that the body

doesn't deliver sufficient insulin or in light of the fact that the cells

don't answer the insulin that is created. This prompts a scope of

intricacies over the long run, including harm to the eyes, kidneys,

nerves, and heart.

In this book, we will investigate the various kinds of diabetes, their

causes and side effects, as well as the different treatment choices accessible. We will likewise examine how to deal with the sickness

through diet, work out, and other way of life changes.

<u>***Section 2***</u>: Kinds of Diabetes

There are three primary kinds of diabetes: type 1, type 2, and

gestational diabetes.

Type 1 diabetes is an immune system sickness where the body's safe

framework assaults and obliterates the cells in the pancreas that

produce insulin. This implies that individuals with type 1 diabetes can't

create insulin and should depend on insulin infusions to direct their

glucose levels.

Type 2 diabetes is the most well-known type of diabetes and happens

when the body becomes impervious to insulin, or doesn't create

sufficient insulin to address its issues. This sort of diabetes is frequently connected to corpulence and a stationary way of life, and can

frequently be overseen through diet and exercise, as well as drug and

insulin treatment.

Gestational diabetes happens during pregnancy and for the most part

disappears after the child is conceived. In any case, ladies who have had

gestational diabetes are at an expanded gamble of creating type 2

diabetes further down the road.

<u>**Section 3**</u>: Causes and Chance Elements

The specific reason for diabetes isn't completely perceived, yet there

are a few factors that can expand the gamble of fostering the sickness.

These include:

- Hereditary qualities: Individuals with a family background of

diabetes are bound to foster the actual infection.

- Corpulence: Being overweight or fat is a significant gamble factor

for type 2 diabetes.

- Stationary way of life: Absence of active work can build the

gamble of creating type 2 diabetes.

- Age: The gamble of creating diabetes increments as we age.

- Nationality: Individuals of specific ethnic foundations, like African Americans, Hispanic/Latinos, and Local Americans, are at a higher gamble of creating diabetes.

Section 4: Side effects and Determination

The side effects of diabetes can differ contingent upon the sort of

diabetes and the person. A few normal side effects include:

- Regular pee

- Expanded thirst

- Unexplained weight reduction

- Weariness

- Obscured vision

- Slow-mending wounds

- Shivering or deadness in the hands or feet

Diabetes can be analyzed through various tests, including a fasting

blood glucose test, an oral glucose resistance test, or a glycated

hemoglobin (A1C) test.

- Diabetes can prompt a scope of complexities over the long run, including nerve harm, kidney sickness, visual deficiency, and cardiovascular illness.

- Diabetic neuropathy is a kind of nerve harm that can cause shivering, deadness, and torment in the hands and feet. It can likewise prompt issues with processing, bladder control, and sexual capability.

- Diabetic retinopathy is a condition that can make harm the veins in the eyes, prompting vision misfortune and visual deficiency.

- Diabetes is likewise a significant gamble factor for cardiovascular illness, including coronary episode and stroke. Elevated degrees of glucose in the blood can harm veins and increment the gamble of

atherosclerosis, a condition in which greasy stores develop in the

supply routes.

<u>**Section 6**</u>: Diabetes and Psychological well-being

- Living with diabetes can likewise essentially affect psychological well-being. The pressure of dealing with the illness, apprehension about inconveniences, and sensations of separation and disgrace can all add to uneasiness and sadness.

- Diabetes is additionally connected with an expanded gamble of dietary problems, especially in young ladies with type 1 diabetes.

- Medical services experts really must evaluate for and address psychological wellness worries in individuals with diabetes, and to give assets and backing to dealing with the close to home parts of the sickness.

<u>**Section 7**</u>: Diabetes and Innovation

- Progresses in innovation are impacting how diabetes is overseen and observed. Constant glucose observing (CGM) frameworks take into account continuous checking of blood glucose levels, while insulin siphons offer more exact conveyance of insulin.

- Fake pancreas frameworks, which join CGM and insulin siphon innovation, are likewise being created to give robotized insulin conveyance and further develop glucose control.

- Portable applications and online stages can likewise assist people with diabetes track their glucose levels, screen their eating regimen and exercise, and interface with medical services experts.

Section 8: Diabetes and Society

- Diabetes is a significant general medical problem that has huge

financial and social effects. The expense of treating diabetes and its

confusions is high, and the infection can likewise prompt loss of

efficiency and decreased personal satisfaction.

- Shame and victimization individuals with diabetes can likewise

add to negative wellbeing results and make it more challenging for

people to deal with the sickness.

- Arrangements and projects that advance diabetes avoidance and the board, as well as drives to decrease shame and separation, are significant for further developing results for individuals with diabetes and lessening the general weight of the infection on society.

<u>**Section 9**</u>: Anticipation:

Forestalling diabetes is a significant stage in lessening the general weight of the illness. While some gamble factors for diabetes, like family ancestry and age, can't be changed, there are a few way of life factors that can be adjusted to diminish the gamble of fostering the sickness. Here are a few ways to forestall diabetes:

1.   Maintain a solid weight: Being overweight or large is a significant gamble factor for type 2 diabetes. Keeping a solid load through normal activity and a decent eating regimen can assist with diminishing the gamble of fostering the infection.

2.   Eat a solid eating regimen: Eating an eating routine that is wealthy

in natural products, vegetables, entire grains, and lean protein sources

can assist with decreasing the gamble of diabetes. Restricting utilization

of handled and sweet food sources can likewise be advantageous.

3.   Exercise consistently: Customary active work can assist with

further developing insulin responsiveness and glucose control, which

can decrease the gamble of diabetes. Hold back nothing 30 minutes of

moderate activity, like lively strolling or cycling, most days of the week.

4.   Quit smoking: Smoking is a gamble factor for the vast majority

persistent infections, including diabetes. Stopping smoking can assist with decreasing the gamble of diabetes and work on generally

wellbeing.

5.   Monitor glucose levels: On the off chance that you have a family

background of diabetes or other gamble factors, it is essential to screen

your glucose levels consistently. This can help distinguish prediabetes

or diabetes early, when way of life changes might be viable in

forestalling or postponing the beginning of the illness.

6.   Manage pressure: Ongoing pressure can add to the improvement

of diabetes. Tracking down ways of overseeing pressure, like through

contemplation, yoga, or other unwinding strategies, can be valuable.

Notwithstanding these way of life factors, a few drugs and mediations

may likewise be successful in forestalling or postponing the beginning

of diabetes. It means a lot to converse with your medical services

supplier about your gamble of diabetes and the best procedures for

counteraction.

<u>**_Section 10_**</u>: Treatment Choices Be that as it may, the sickness can be

successfully made do with the right therapy and way of life changes.

Here are the absolute most ideal ways to treat diabetes:

1.   Medications: There are a few prescriptions accessible to assist

with overseeing diabetes, including insulin and oral meds that can assist

with directing glucose levels. Your medical care supplier can assist with

figuring out which medicine or mix of prescriptions is ideal for you.

2.   Blood sugar observing: Checking your glucose levels routinely is a

significant piece of overseeing diabetes. This can assist you with

recognizing patterns and make acclimations to your treatment plan

depending on the situation.

3.   Healthy eating: A solid eating routine is a critical part of

overseeing diabetes. Eating an eating regimen that is wealthy in natural

products, vegetables, entire grains, and lean protein sources, and

restricting handled and sweet food sources can assist with controlling

glucose levels and work on generally wellbeing.

4.   Regular activity: Normal activity can assist with further developing

insulin responsiveness and glucose control, which can lessen the

gamble of complexities related with diabetes. Hold back nothing 30

minutes of moderate activity most days of the week.

5.   Weight administration: Keeping a sound weight can assist with

further developing glucose control and lessen the gamble of difficulties

related with diabetes.

6.   Stress the executives: Persistent pressure can add to the turn of

events and deteriorating of diabetes. Tracking down ways of overseeing

pressure, like through reflection, yoga, or other unwinding strategies,

can be gainful.

7.   Regular clinical check-ups: Ordinary check-ups with your medical

care supplier can help recognize and deal with any difficulties related

with diabetes, for example, kidney illness, nerve harm, and eye issues.

It is vital to work intimately with your medical services supplier to

foster a far reaching care plan that is customized to your singular

requirements and objectives. With appropriate administration and

care, people with diabetes can have full and dynamic existences.

Section 11: Overseeing Diabetes

Living with diabetes requires cautious administration to forestall

difficulties and keep up with great wellbeing. This incorporates

observing glucose levels consistently, following a sound eating regimen,

getting standard activity, and accepting drugs as recommended.

It's additionally critical to know about the signs and side effects of

complexities, like neuropathy, retinopathy, and cardiovascular illness,

<u>**_Section 12_**</u>: Living with Diabetes

- Living with diabetes can be testing, however there are numerous assets accessible to assist people with dealing with the illness and keep up with great wellbeing.

- Support gatherings, instructive projects, and online assets can all give significant data and backing to individuals with diabetes.

- Systems for adapting to the profound and mental parts of living with diabetes, for example, stress the executives and care rehearses, can likewise be useful.

<u>**_Section 13_**</u>: Future Turns of events (proceeded)

- Propels in examination and innovation are continually working on how we might interpret diabetes and prompting new medicines and mediations.

- Examination into the utilization of counterfeit pancreas frameworks, immature microorganism treatment, and quality altering innovations shows guarantee for the treatment and possible fix of diabetes.

- New medications and treatments are additionally being created to further develop glucose control and lessen the gamble of intricacies.

<u>**_Section 14:_** End</u>

- Diabetes is a perplexing and testing illness that requires progressing the executives and care. Nonetheless, with the right apparatuses and support, people with diabetes can have full and dynamic existences.

- Progresses in examination and innovation are working on how we might interpret diabetes and prompting new medicines and mediations. People with diabetes genuinely must remain informed about new turns of events and to work with their medical services group to foster an extensive consideration plan.

- Diabetes is likewise a general medical problem with huge monetary and social effects. Tending to the underlying drivers of the illness, advancing avoidance and early mediation, and decreasing shame and segregation are immensely significant for further developing results and diminishing the general weight of diabetes on society.